USMLE Step 2 (**Quick Notes**)
Dermatology

- The most comprehensive and up-to-date high yield review available for the USMLE® Step 2 CK
- Easy-to-follow illustrated quick review for the most critical facts of the USMLE Examination.
- Uses effective learning tools, from key facts and mnemonics to full-color images and illustrations.
- Written by Dr. Tarek Abdelhamid (Dr. Tarek*) who is the first person to successfully integrate effective learning models into the field of Medical Education (See: Dr. Tarek's ground-breaking medical educational model: **The Multidimensional Learning Model** [Tarek's Integrated System for Learning and Memory]).

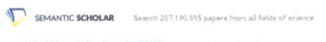

The Multidimensional Learning Model: A Novel Cognitive Psychology-Based Model for Computer Assisted Instruction in Order to Improve Learning in Medical Students

Tarek Abdelhamid · Published 9 December 1999 · Psychology · Medical Education Online

Copyright © 2023 by Dr. Tarek Abdelhamid M.D.
All rights reserved. No part of this publication may be reproduced, distributed, or transmitted in any form or by any means, including photocopying, recording, or other electronic or mechanical methods, without the prior written permission of the author.

Special thanks to Dr. Maha Atout

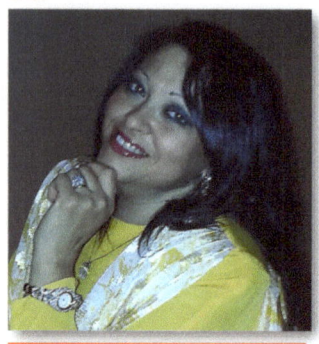

Dr. Maha Atout M.D.

Special thanks to my dear wife Dr. Maha Atout M.D. for her great educational contributions to this book and to all my life.
Dr. Tarek Abdelhamid

Contents

1.	Acne Vulgaris	5
2.	Rosacea	10
3.	Hidradenitis Suppurativa	13
4.	Atopic Dermatitis (Eczema)	15
5.	Contact Dermatitis	17
6.	Psoriasis	21
7.	Seborrheic Dermatitis	25
8.	Pityriasis Rosea	27
9.	Lichen Planus	29
10.	Urticaria (Hives)	30
11.	Angioedema	32
12.	Anaphylaxis	35
13.	Drug Reactions	38
14.	Erythema Multiforme	43
15.	Stevens-Johnson Syndrome	45
16.	Erythroderma	48
17.	Erythema Nodosum	49
18.	Pyoderma Gangrenosum	51
19.	Bullous Pemphigoid	53

20.	Pemphigus Vulgaris	54
21.	Vitiligo	56
22.	Impetigo	57
23.	Skin Abscess	58
24.	Cellulitus	59
25.	Necrotizing Fasciitis	61
26.	Warts	62
27.	Molluscum Contagiosum	66
28.	Herpes Zoster (Shingles)	68
29.	Dermatophytes	72
30.	Tinea Versicolor	76
31.	Scabies	78
32.	Actinic Keratosis	81
33.	Seborrheic Keratosis	83
34.	Keratoacanthoma	85
35.	Basal Cell Carcinoma	86
36.	Squamous Cell Carcinoma (SCC)	87
37.	Melanoma	88

1 Acne Vulgaris

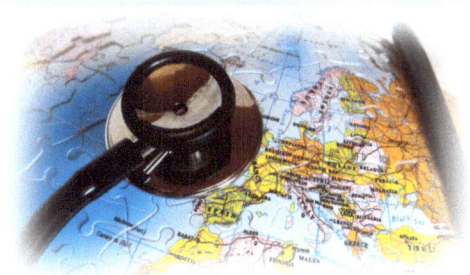

Acne Vulgaris

Acne Vulgaris is an inflammatory condition of the skin that is most prevalent during adolescence.

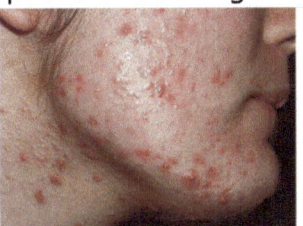

Risk factors are male sex, puberty, Cushing syndrome, oily complexion, excess androgens, and medications.

There is no proven link between acne and diet (e.g., chocolate, fatty foods).

Acne Vulgaris

Pathogenesis of Acne Vulgaris:
1) Follicular hyperkeratinization.
2) Increased sebum production.
3) Obstruction of sebaceous follicles (by sebum) leading to the proliferation of Cutibacterium acnes (an anaerobic bacterium, formerly known as Propionibacterium acnes).
4) Inflammation as a result of C. acnes proliferation.

Cutibacterium acnes is an anaerobic bacterium, formerly known as Propionibacterium acnes.

Acne Vulgaris

XXXXXX

Types:
1) Obstructive: open comedones (blackheads) or closed comedones (whiteheads).

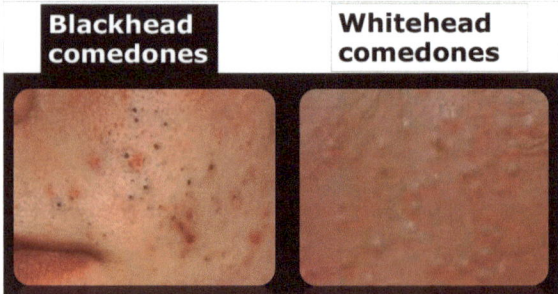

| Blackhead comedones | Whitehead comedones |

Acne Vulgaris

Treatment: General guidelines:
1) Instruct patient to keep affected area clean (Regular washing)
2) Reduce or discontinue acne-promoting agents (certain make-up, creams, oils, steroids, androgens).

Use of Medications

Note: It takes about 6 weeks to notice the effects of medications (In fact, skin may get worse before it gets better). Start with one drug to assess its efficacy.

Acne Vulgaris

Medical Treatment (Step 1):
Mild Acne
Begin with topical benzoyl peroxide (2.5%)—should be applied once or twice daily. It destroys acne-causing bacteria and prevents plugging of pores by drying the skin.

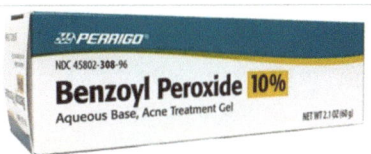

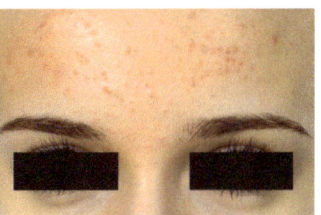

Acne Vulgaris

Medical Treatment (Step 2): Moderate Acne

1) Add Topical Retinoids if benzoyl peroxide (2.5%) failed. They cause peeling of the skin, which prevents clogging of pores.

2) Add Topical Erythromycin or Topical Clindamycin—both act to suppress C. acnes.

Start with one drug to assess its efficacy.

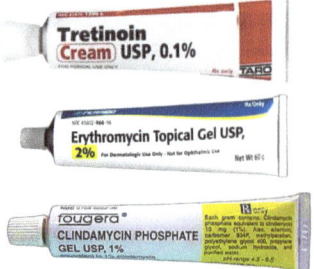

Acne Vulgaris

Medical Treatment (Step 3): Severe Acne
Nodular pustular acne

1) Add systemic antibiotic therapy: tetracycline, doxycycline, erythromycin, clindamycin, azithromycin, and TMP-SMX (Only if previous measures failed).

2) Add oral retinoids (Isotretinoin) for severe, recalcitrant, nodular acne that is not responsive to the above treatments.

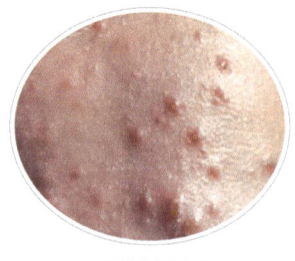

Acne Vulgaris

Note:

Oral retinoids are extremely teratogenic.

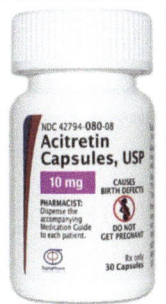

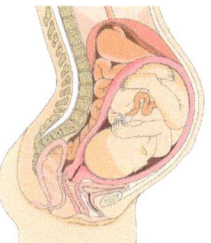

1. All female patients who are going to use **Retinoids** must have two negative pregnancy tests before starting oral Isotretinoin.
2. In addition, they should use two forms of birth control for 1 month **before** starting the medication through 1 month after stopping the medication.

2 Rosacea

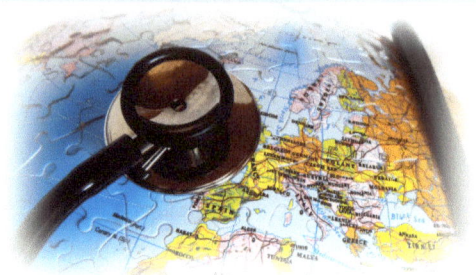

Rosacea

A chronic condition resulting in reddening of the face (mainly the forehead, nose, and cheeks). It often appears very similar to acne, but unlike acne it first starts in middle age.

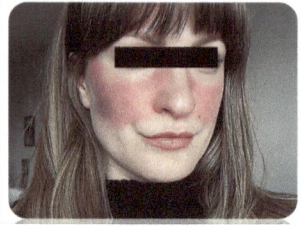

Mostly affects Caucasian women between 30 and 50 years of age.

Rosacea

The most common skin findings of Rosacea are - erythema, telangiectasia, papules, and pustules with redness, typically affecting the face.

Unlike acne vulgaris, there are **No comedones** in Rosacea.

Rhinophyma

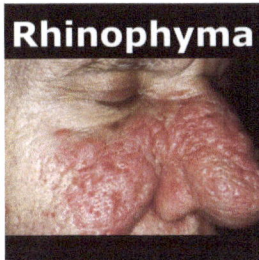

In severe cases of Rosacea skin can become thickened and greasy—On the nose, it creates a bulbous appearance called **Rhinophyma** (mostly seen in men).

Rosacea

❶ Treatment of erythema and flushing:
Avoid alcohol, hot beverages, extremes of temperature, and emotional stressors.
If inadequate, **Topical Brimonidine** can be used.

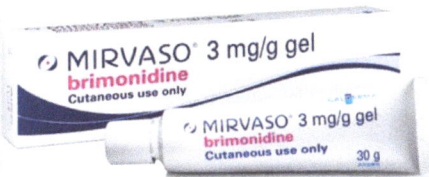

Rosacea

② Treatment of papules and pustules:
1) Start with **Topical Metronidazole** gel (Alternatives are Azelaic acid and Topical Ivermectin).
2) If the above treatment is not adequate, you can add systemic antibiotics such as **Tetracyclines**.
3) If all the above, failed use **Oral Isotretinoin** as a last option.

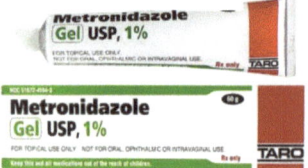

3. Hidradenitis Suppurativa

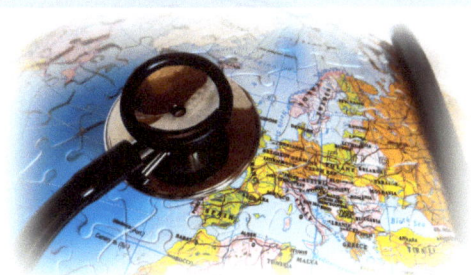

Hidradenitis Suppurativa

Inflammatory skin condition affecting intertriginous areas (**axilla is the most common site**), causing nodules, abscesses, and draining sinus tracts that can result in scarring.
More common in **women**
Typical onset in second or third decade of life.
Strong relationship with smoking.

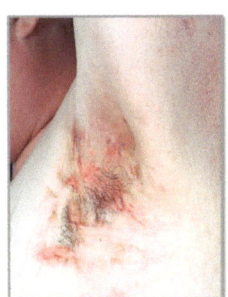

Hidradenitis Suppurativa

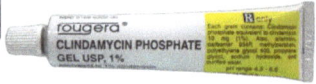

Treatment
1) For **Mild** disease, **Topical** Clindamycin may be used.
2) For **Moderate** disease, **Oral** antibiotics, oral retinoids, or hormonal therapy may be used. If the response is unsatisfactory, adalimumab may be used.
3) For **Severe** extensive disease, surgical excision is often required.

4. Atopic Dermatitis (Eczema)

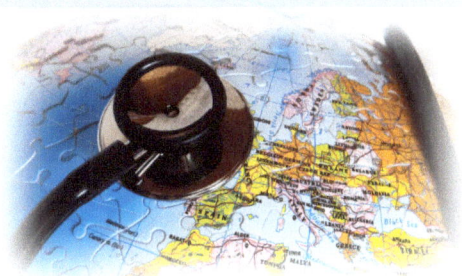

Atopic Dermatitis (Eczema)

Eczema is more frequent in children but also occurs in adults. Commonly involves flexor surfaces (e.g., antecubital and popliteal fossae, wrists).

Commonly associated with a personal or family history of atopy (such as seasonal allergies, bronchial asthma).

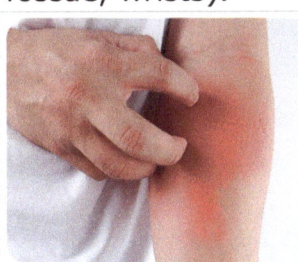

Atopic Dermatitis (Eczema)

Treatment:
1) **Eliminate triggers** (allergens, frequent bathing without moisturizing, heat, low humidity)
2) **Use adjuncts** such as antihistamines for pruritus.
3) **Topical steroids** should be used for affected areas, with the potency of steroids chosen based on severity.

Topical calcineurin inhibitors (Tacrolimus) can be used if there is an inadequate response to high potency steroids.

Topical steroids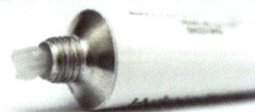

5 Contact Dermatitis

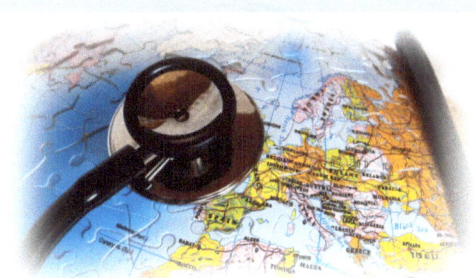

Contact Dermatitis

There are two forms of contact dermatitis:

(1) Irritant contact dermatitis is more common and results from a chemical or physical insult to the skin (Contact with detergents, acids, or alkalis, or from frequent hand washing). It is not an immunologic reaction).

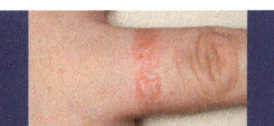

The rash begins shortly after exposure to the irritant (in contrast to the allergic type, which begins several hours to a few days later).

Contact Dermatitis

(2) Allergic contact dermatitis is a delayed-type hypersensitivity (type IV) reaction.

Sensitization of the skin occurs 1 to 2 weeks after the first exposure to the allergen. Subsequent exposure leads to dermatitis hours to days after the reexposure.

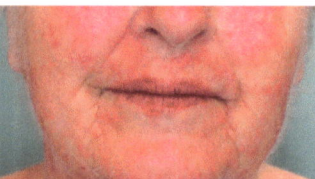

No history of atopy is necessary for allergic contact dermatitis to occur.

Common allergens include poison ivy, oak, and sumac; iodine; nickel; rubber; topical medications; and cosmetics.

Contact Dermatitis

The appearance of the rash depends on the stage.

❶ **Acute stage:** erythematous papules and vesicles with oozing edema may be present.

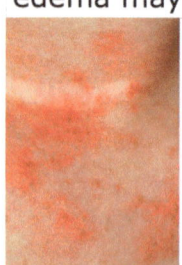 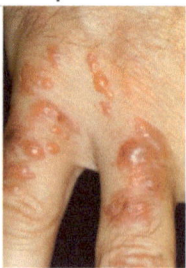

Contact Dermatitis

The appearance of the rash depends on the stage.
② **Chronic stage:** crusting, thickening, and scaling; lichenification.
The rash is usually very pruritic and is found only in exposed areas.
The interval between exposure and appearance of the rash varies, but is usually from several hours to as long as 4 to 5 days.

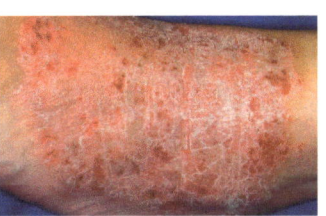

Contact Dermatitis

Diagnosis is usually made clinically based on history and examination.

Patch testing (to identify the allergen that caused the allergic reaction). It is indicated if the diagnosis is in doubt, the rash does not respond to treatment, or the rash recurs.

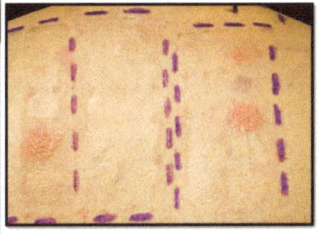

Contact Dermatitis

Treatment
Avoid the contact allergen!
Apply cool tap water compresses.
Apply topical corticosteroids.

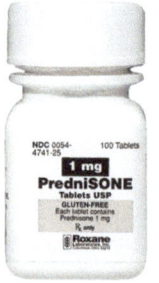

If the case is severe, prescribe systemic corticosteroids (Such as prednisone, 1 mg/kg/day).

Continue systemic corticosteroids for 10 to 14 days and then reduce the dose gradually.

Contact Dermatitis

Do not confuse allergic contact dermatitis with any of the following:

1) **Irritant contact dermatitis**—Rash begins very soon after exposure
2) **Atopic dermatitis**—Onset is in infancy or childhood
3) **Seborrheic dermatitis** Common in scalp, upper chest, and back
4) **Psoriasis-** Plaques covered with scales. elbows, knees, lower back and scalp

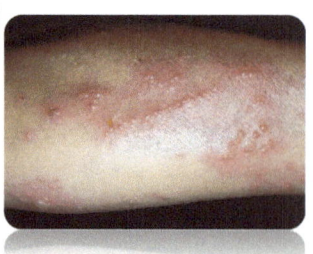

6 Psoriasis

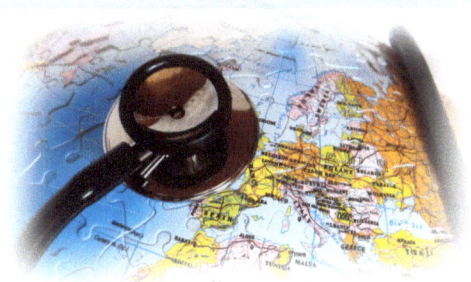

Psoriasis

1) A chronic condition characterized by exacerbations and remissions—it improves during the summer (sun exposure) and worsens in the winter (dries skin).
2) injury(Koebner phenomenon).
3) Up to three-fourths of patients have localized disease (<20% to 25% of body surface area [BSA]).

Less than 10% of patients develop psoriatic arthritis

Psoriasis

Clinical Manifestations
The most common clinical subtype is chronic plaque psoriasis.
Lesions are well-demarcated, erythematous papules or **plaques** that are covered by thick, silvery scaling; pruritus is rarely present.
It can involve any part of the body, but the most common areas are the **extensor surfaces** of extremities (knees, elbows), scalp, intergluteal cleft, palms, and soles.

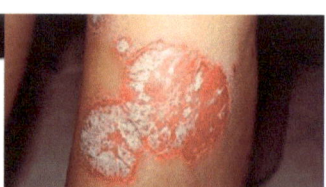

Psoriasis

Pitting of the nails or Onycholysis (Distal separation of the nail from the nail bed).

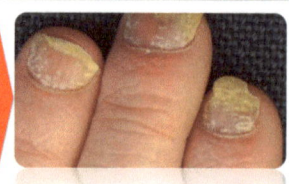

Auspitz sign—removal of the scale causes pinpoint bleeding.

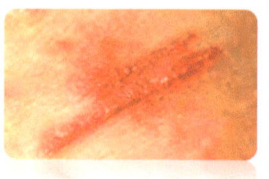

Psoriasis

Treatment: Topical therapy
Corticosteroids and emollients are the most commonly prescribed first-line agents.

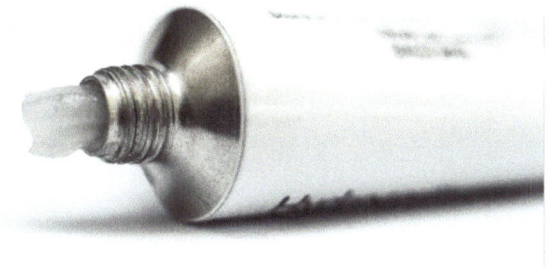

Psoriasis

Treatment: Topical therapy
Calcipotriene and calcitriol are **vitamin D derivatives** that have become first- Or second-line agents in treating psoriasis. They are very effective in most patients.

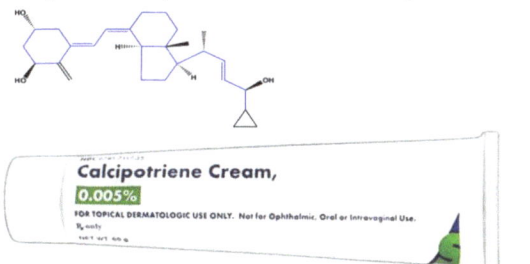

Psoriasis

Treatment: Topical therapy
Tars have unpleasant odor, so they are less desirable to use. Patients should use tars for 4 to 6 weeks before expecting to see a benefit. Tars are more effective in combination therapy and are associated with an 80% to 90% remission rate.

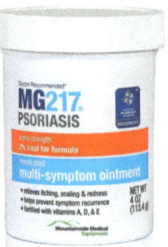

Note 1: Combination therapy (steroids + calcipotriene) is more effective than either agent alone.

Note 2: Phototherapy (with ultraviolet light) should be used for moderate–severe psoriasis if feasible.

Psoriasis

Systemic treatment of Psoriasis is indicated in patients with severe psoriasis.

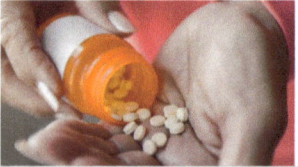

1) Immune-modulating therapy (Methotrexate, Cyclosporine Infliximab)
2) Oral retinoids (e.g., acitretin)
3) Combinations of these agents with phototherapy.

Note: Oral steroids should be avoided in psoriasis
As discontinuation can cause flaring and can precipitate erythroderma.

7 Seborrheic Dermatitis

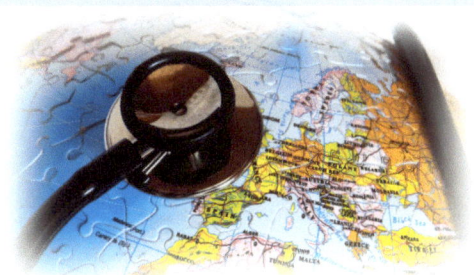

Seborrheic Dermatitis

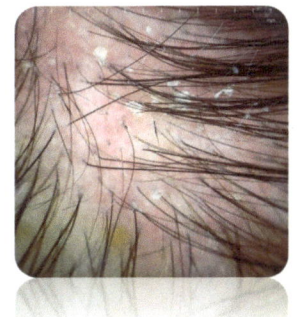

A very **common** chronic, idiopathic, inflammatory skin disorder that occurs in all age groups (affects 5% of the population).
More common in patients with oily skin.

Exacerbating factors include - anxiety, stress, fatigue, hormonal factors.

| Pruritus, skin lesions, and hair loss can occur if left untreated. | May be complicated by secondary bacterial infection. |

Seborrheic Dermatitis

Manifestations:
1) Dandruff
2) Yellowish, oily, and thick flakes that appear near eyelashes, in the ear canal, on the middle chest, behind the ears, and other skin folds.
3) Scaly patches with surrounding areas of mild to moderate erythema.

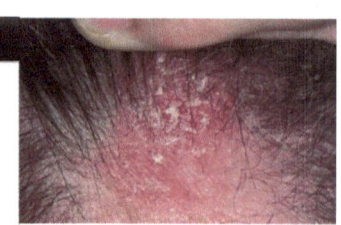

Seborrheic Dermatitis

Treatment
1) **Sunlight** exposure often helps.
2) **Dandruff shampoo** (over-the-counter) is usually adequate.
3) **Topical ketoconazole** (to decrease yeast count on skin) has been found to be effective.
4) **Topical corticosteroids** for severe cases.

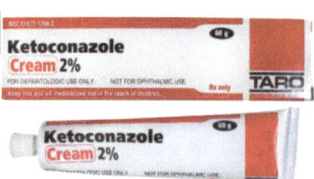

8 Pityriasis Rosea

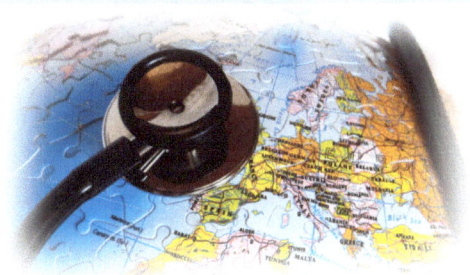

Pityriasis Rosea

Papulosquamous eruption—Initially, "herald patches" (Multiple round/oval patches) appear, and then a generalized rash with multiple oval-shaped lesions appears. The **rash** is classically described as having a **Christmas tree**-appearance.

It is not contagious and is possibly related to herpes type 7.

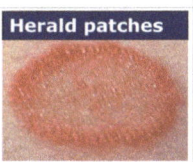

Herald patches

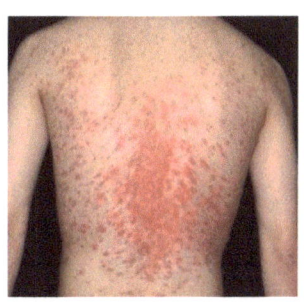

Pityriasis Rosea

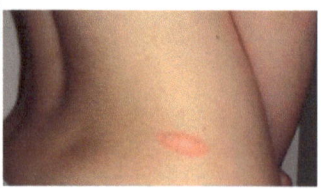

1) It is **common on** the trunk and upper arms and thighs and is usually not found on the face.
2) Pruritus is often present and varies in severity.
3) It spontaneously remits within a few (6 to 8) weeks without treatment.

Treatment is antihistamines for pruritus.

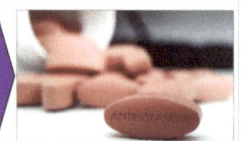

9 Lichen Planus

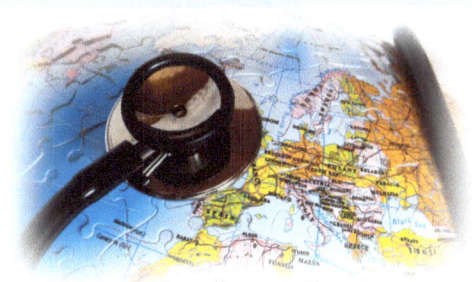

Lichen Planus

1) Chronic, inflammatory mucocutaneous lesions of unknown etiology.
2) It may be associated with hepatitis C and certain drugs.
3) It is characterized by : **P**ruritic, **P**olygonal, **P**urple, flat-topped **P**apules.
4) Most commonly seen on wrists, shins, oral mucosa, and genitalia.
5) Treat with steroids.

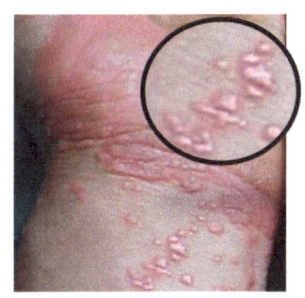

10 Urticaria (Hives)

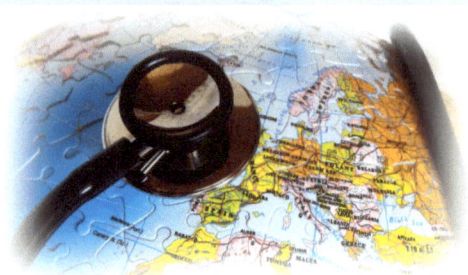

Urticaria (Hives)

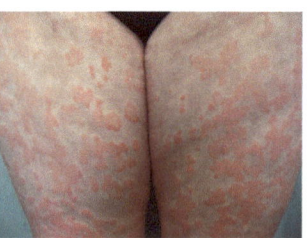

Urticaria is an allergic condition triggered by different allergens such as food, drugs, animal dander, pollen, dust, plants, or infections.

Findings—Migratory edematous wheals (hives) that often quickly appear and then disappear. They blanch with pressure and may cause intense pruritus or stinging. Lesions get worse with scratching

Urticaria (Hives)

Treatment involves removal of the offending agent. Antihistamines are effective for symptomatic relief. Systemic corticosteroids may help in more severe cases.

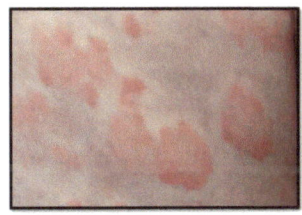
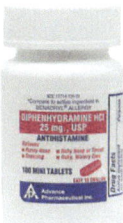
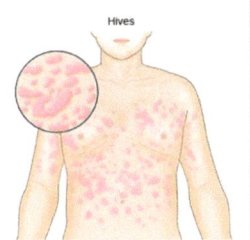

Urticaria (Hives)

Unlike erythema multiforme, urticaria has a clear or pink center and is blanchable.

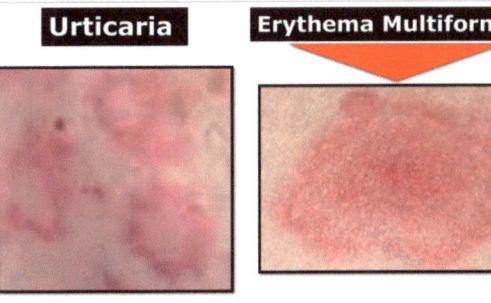

11 Angioedema

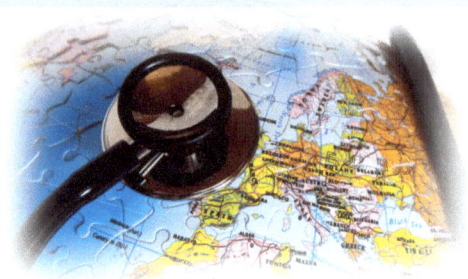

Angioedema

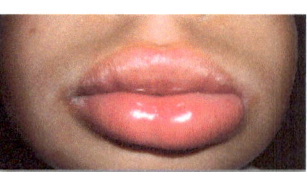

1) **Angioedema** is an allergic reaction that can be caused by any of the precipitants of urticaria.
2) **ACE inhibitors** are a specific cause of angioedema (**Note:** Reaction in this situation usually occurs within 1 week of initiating the drug).
3) **Unlike urticaria**, which can occur anywhere, angioedema usually affects the eyelids, lips and tongue, genitalia, hands, or feet.

Angioedema

\# Angioedema results in nonpitting, puffy skin with firm swelling that is **more tender (or "burning") than pruritic** (due to less mast cells and nerve endings in deeper tissues).
\# Angioedema can involve the GI tract, causing nausea/vomiting and abdominal pain (**Can mimic acute abdomen**).
\# Severe angioedema can lead to potentially **life-threatening airway obstruction**.

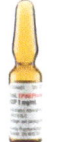

Give SC epinephrine for laryngeal edema or bronchospasm.

Treatment is similar to treatment of urticaria.

Angioedema

Note: Hereditary angioedema: autosomal dominant condition caused by **C1 esterase inhibitor deficiency**, characterized by recurrent episodes of angioedema; can be life-threatening

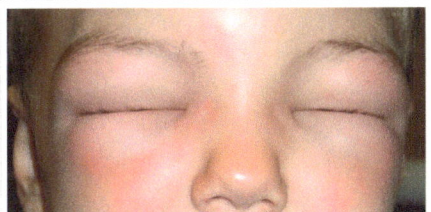

Angioedema
Hereditary angioedema

Ecallantide, a recombinant protein that acts as a reversible inhibitor of kallikrein, is currently indicated for acute attacks of HAE in those aged ≥12 years.

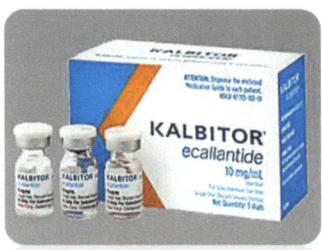

Angioedema
Hereditary angioedema

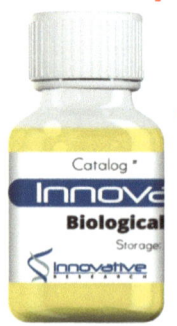

Purified plasma-derived human C1 esterase inhibitor concentrate is the treatment of choice for short-term prophylaxis.

Tranexamic acid and Danazol can be used for long-term prophylaxis.

12 Anaphylaxis

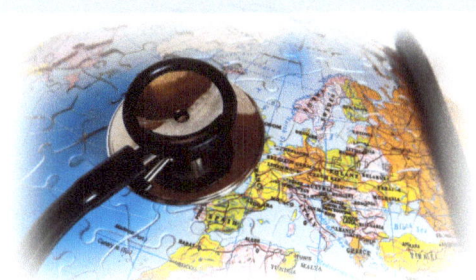

Anaphylaxis

1) A **life-threatening** systemic allergic reaction caused by a massive release of mast cell mediators (usually a type I hypersensitivity reaction) that
2) Occurs within **seconds to minutes** of exposure to an allergen.
3) **Numerous allergens have been identified**. These include foods (Most common cause), medications, radiocontrast agents, blood products, venoms (e.g., from snakes), insect stings, latex, hormones, ragweed/molds, and several chemicals.

Anaphylaxis

Clinical findings include
1) **Skin and mucosal signs** (most common and early findings urticaria, swollen lips and tongue, periorbital edema)
2) **Respiratory signs** (dyspnea, wheeze, airway obstruction)
3) **GI signs** (nausea/vomiting, crampy abdominal pain)
4) **Cardiovascular signs** (tachycardia, hypotension, shock)

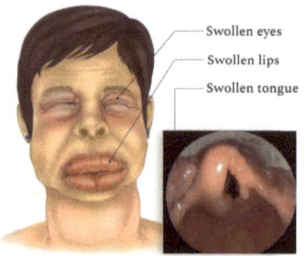

Anaphylaxis

Treatment of anaphylaxis:
ABCs—secure the airway (intubation may be necessary) and provide supplemental oxygen, treat hypotension with rapid infusion of IV fluids.

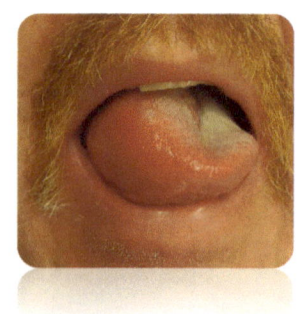

Anaphylaxis

Treatment of anaphylaxis:
Give **IM epinephrine** immediately; may require several doses of 0.3 to 0.5 mg (1 mg/mL preparation). If not responding, prepare IV epinephrine infusion.

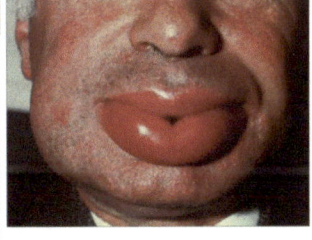

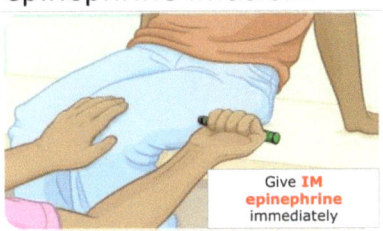

Give **IM epinephrine** immediately

Anaphylaxis

Treatment of anaphylaxis:
If still wheezing despite epinephrine, give **albuterol** for bronchospasm.

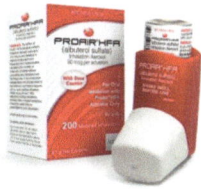

Adjuncts to treatment may include: antihistamines (both H1 and H2 blockers such as diphenhydramine and ranitidine) and corticosteroids.

13 Drug Reactions

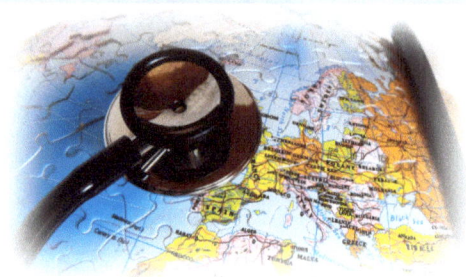

Drug Reactions (General)

1) β-Lactam antibiotics (penicillins), aspirin, NSAIDs, and sulfa drugs account for more than 80% of all cases of drug allergy.
2) Drug-induced hypersensitivity reactions most commonly manifest as type IV reactions with diffuse maculopapular eruptions
3) Can affect multiple organ systems (Skin, Interstitial nephritis, pneumonitis, Cardiovascular collapse anaphylaxis, etc.).

Note 1: Allergic drug reactions reactions typically appear within 1 month of initiating the drug.

Note 2: It is uncommon for a drug reaction to occur within less than 1 week of initiating the drug.

Fixed Drug Eruption

Fixed Drug Eruption
1) Typically caused by antibiotics or NSAIDs
2) Appears early (within hours) after reexposure to the precipitating medication in the same body location.
3) A purple patch(s) will typically appear. The lesions typically resolve spontaneously, leaving an area of post-inflammatory hyperpigmentation.

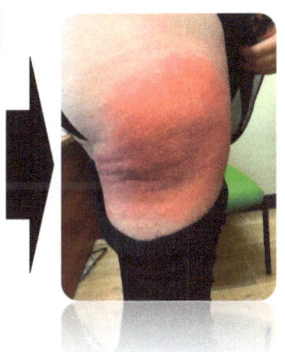

Types of Hypersensitivity Reactions

Type I: IgE-mediated (anaphylaxis, asthma)
Type II: IgG- (or IgM-) and cytotoxic cell-mediated (Goodpasture disease, pemphigus vulgaris)
Type III: antigen–antibody complexes (SLE, Arthus reaction, serum sickness)
Type IV: T-cell–mediated (delayed hypersensitivity) (e.g., allergic contact dermatitis, tuberculosis, transplant rejection)

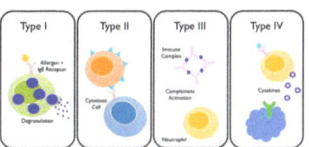

Acute Generalized Exanthematous Pustulosis (AGEP)

1) AGEP presents with fever, leukocytosis, and a skin eruption of small pustules on an erythematous background.
2) AGEP eruption typically occurs within hours or days after exposure to the drug, and typically begins on the face and neck and then spreads to the trunk and limbs.
3) Antibiotics are the most common culprit, and treatment is supportive.
4) Treat by discontinuing the medication and topical steroids.

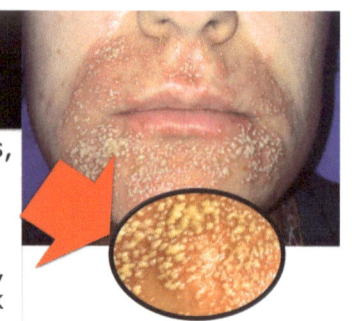

Drug Reaction With Eosinophilia and Systemic Symptoms (DRESS)

A systemic reaction that typically occurs 2 to 6 weeks after starting a medication (longer latency than other drug reactions).
Initial symptoms include fever, lymphadenopathy, facial edema, and a diffuse, morbilliform skin eruption.

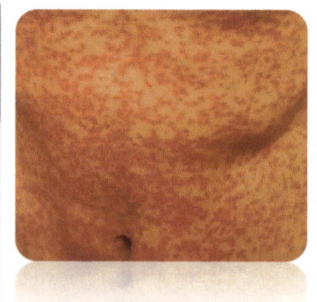

Drug Reaction With Eosinophilia and Systemic Symptoms (DRESS)

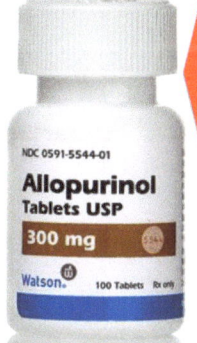

The most common precipitating medications are allopurinol, antiepileptics, and sulfa drugs.

Drug Reaction With Eosinophilia and Systemic Symptoms (DRESS)

Diagnosis is made using a clinical scoring system based on:
(1) History of exposure to a common medication
(2) Typical examination findings (Fever, morbilliform eruption)
(3) Laboratory abnormalities (Eosinophilia, abnormal liver enzymes, acute kidney injury).

The reaction can progress to involve multiple organ systems, most commonly the liver, kidneys, and lung.

Drug Reaction With Eosinophilia and Systemic Symptoms (DRESS)

1) Withdraw the offending agent
2) Use steroids if there is significant lung or kidney or Liver involvement.

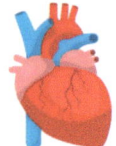 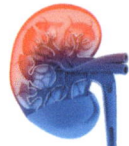 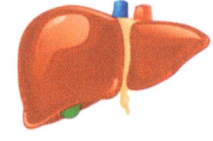

Liver involvement can sometimes progress to acute liver failure requiring transplant.

14 Erythema Multiforme

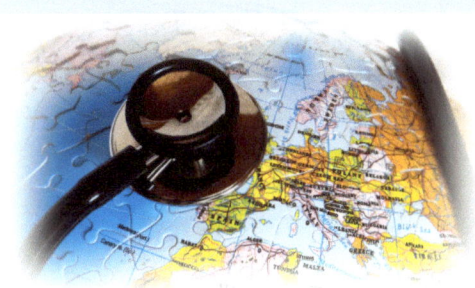

Erythema Multiforme

Erythema multiforme (EM) is an inflammatory skin condition characterized by erythematous macules/papules that resemble target lesions ("bull's-eye lesions") that can become bullous).

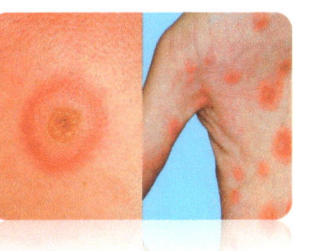

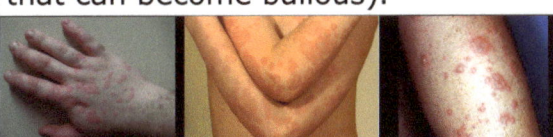

Skin lesions may be pruritic and painful, and often affect the palms, soles, and mouth.

Erythema Multiforme

1) Erythema Multiforme can be caused by infections and medications.
2) EM is caused by infection in 90% of cases. Viral, bacterial, and fungal infections particularly HSV and Mycoplasma.
3) The most common precipitating medications are antibiotics, sulfa drugs, antiepileptics, and NSAIDs.

Other causes of EM include autoimmune disease, malignancy, vaccines, and radiation.

Erythema Multiforme

Treatment is directed at the underlying etiology (Acyclovir for HSV).
Topical steroids and oral antihistamines are used for symptomatic relief
Oral steroids can be used for more severe cases.

15 Stevens–Johnson Syndrome

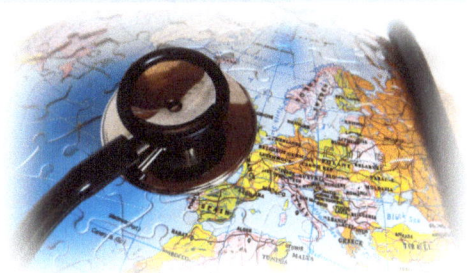

Stevens–Johnson Syndrome

Stevens–Johnson Syndrome (SJS) and Toxic Epidermal Necrolysis (TEN) are part of a disease continuum of severe mucocutaneous eruptions.

SIS and TEN are Dermatologic Emergencies.

SJS involves <10% BSA, and TEN involves >30% BSA.

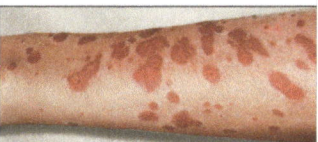

Note: The "rule of nines" is the quickest method of estimating the affected BSA—the head is 9%, each arm is 9%, each leg is 18%, and each side of the trunk (anterior and posterior) is 18%

Stevens–Johnson Syndrome

1) The **majority** of cases of SJS are caused by medications (most commonly antiepileptics, sulfa antibiotics, allopurinol, nevirapine, and NSAIDs),
2) One third (1/3) of the cases have no apparent trigger.
3) Mycoplasma is a known infectious precipitant.

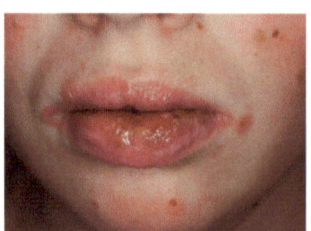

Stevens–Johnson Syndrome

Skin lesions are typically coalescing erythematous macules and **target lesions** that progress to vesicles/bullae with extensive skin necrosis and sloughing.

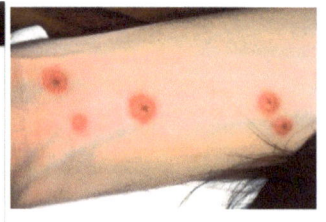

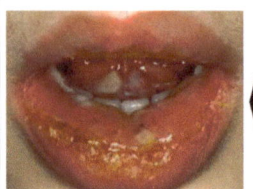

Mucosal involvement is very common in both SJS and TEN.

Stevens–Johnson Syndrome

Other complications include massive fluid and electrolyte loss, secondary infections and sepsis, and multiorgan failure.

Mortality rate is 10% for SJS and 30% for TEN

Management:
1. Admit to ICU or burn unit.
2. Withdraw the suspected medication
3. Aggressive rehydration and symptomatic management.
4. Urgent dermatology ophthalmology consultation.

16 Erythroderma

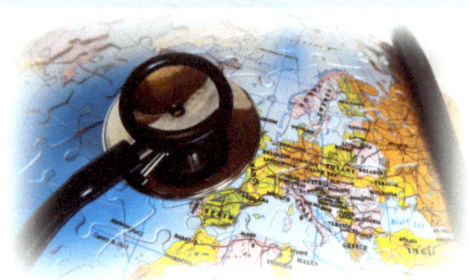

Erythroderma

A **life-threatening** dermatologic emergency that causes erythema and scaling that involves 90% or more of the patient's BSA. It may be **caused by** medications, as a reaction to infection, or a flare of an existing dermatitis (e.g., atopic dermatitis or psoriasis).
Treatment involves intensive skin care (emollients, dressings, warm and humid environment), oral antihistamines and topical steroids, and addressing the underlying condition.

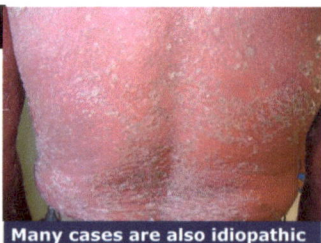
Many cases are also idiopathic

It may occur after abrupt discontinuation of oral steroids.

17 Erythema Nodosum

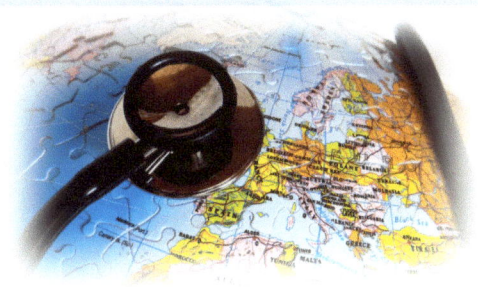

Erythema Nodosum

Erythema nodosum appears as painful, red, subcutaneous, elevated nodules, typically located over the anterior aspect of the tibia.
It may be associated with Low-grade fever, malaise, and joint pain may precede the rash.

Triggers include
- Infections
- Drugs
- Malignancy
- Inflammatory Bowel Disease (IBD)
- Pregnancy

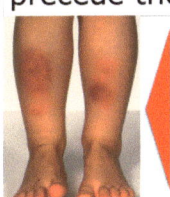

It is much more common in women (especially young women) than in men.

It is self-limited and usually resolves within few weeks.

Erythema Nodosum

Perform the following to help determine the underlying condition:
Chest X-Ray (for sarcoidosis, tuberculosis, other infections)
Antistreptolysin-O titer, CBC, ESR and C-reactive protein
Tuberculin test or interferon-gamma release assay for T.B.

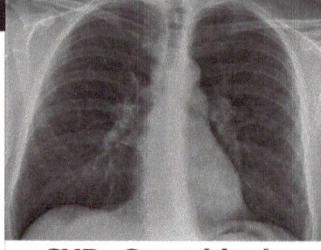

CXR- Sarcoidosis

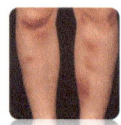

Erythema Nodosum

(1) Treat the underlying condition, if known.
(2) Prescribe bed rest & leg elevation.
(3) NSAIDs, and heat for symptoms.
(4) Potassium iodide may help.

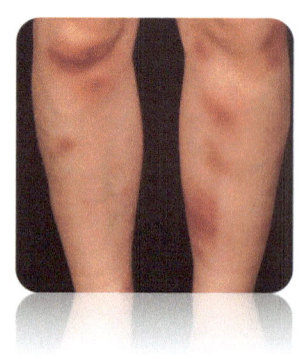

18 Pyoderma Gangrenosum

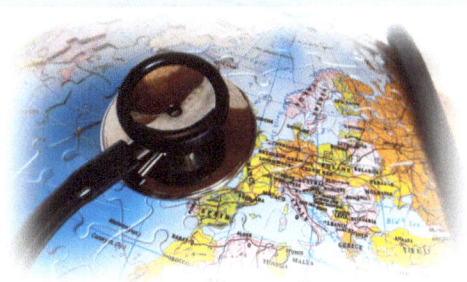

Pyoderma Gangrenosum

Pyoderma Gangrenosum is a neutrophilic dermatosis that most commonly presents with **ulcerating lesions**

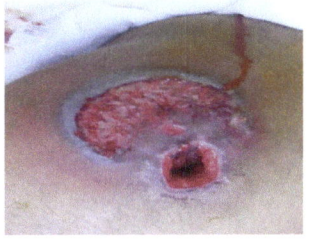

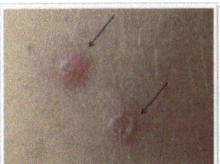

PG can be exacerbated by minor trauma leading to exaggerated skin injury such as Papule, Pustule, Ulceration, a condition known as "pathergy".

Note: Pathergy test is Non- specific test as it can be +ve in: Behçet disease- Pyoderma gangrenosum- Inflammatory bowel disease (IBD)

Pyoderma Gangrenosum

Pyoderma gangrenosum is commonly associated with IBD, hematologic disease (especially IgA monoclonal gammopathy), and rheumatologic disease (such as rheumatoid arthritis)

Pyoderma Gangrenosum

Treatment involves nontraumatic wound care *Plus* topical agents such as high potency steroids or tacrolimus.

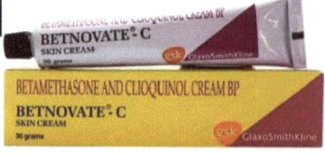

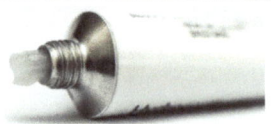

If severe or fails to respond to initial measures, then alternatives include systemic dapsone or minocycline, or immunomodulating therapies such as cyclosporine.

19 Bullous Pemphigoid

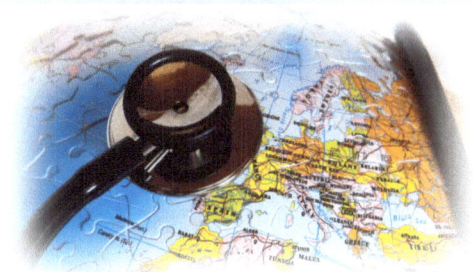

Bullous Pemphigoid

1) Multiple subepithelial blisters on abdomen, groin, and extremities.
2) Elderly people are most affected.
3) Blisters are less easily ruptured than in pemphigus vulgaris.
4) Autoimmune condition
5) No malignant potential but may be persistent.
6) Treat with systemic or topical glucocorticoids.

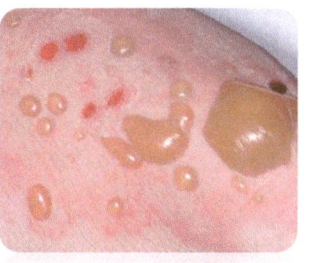

20 Pemphigus Vulgaris

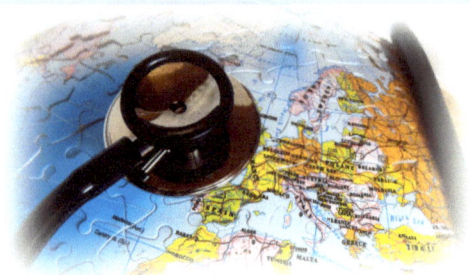

Pemphigus Vulgaris

Autoimmune blistering condition resulting in loss of normal adhesion between cells (acantholysis).
Starts in oral mucosa and may become generalized.
Blisters rupture leaving painful erosions.
Most commonly affects elderly people
Often fatal if untreated.
Treat with systemic glucocorticoids and other immunosuppressants.

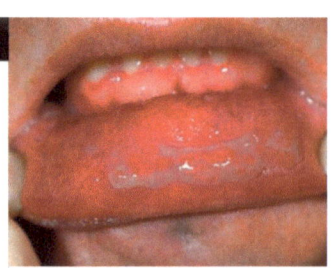

Pemphigus Vulgaris

Note: Pemphigus Vulgaris may be the presenting symptoms of malignancies such as non-Hodgkin lymphoma, chronic lymphocytic leukemia, and Castleman disease.

Associated with Autoantibodies (Usually IgG) directed against the adhesion molecule desmoglein.

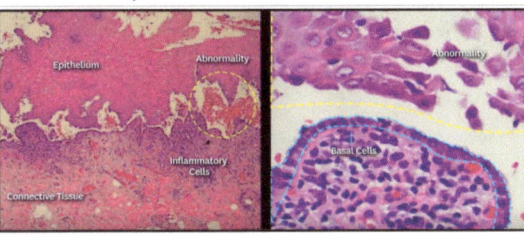

21 | Vitiligo

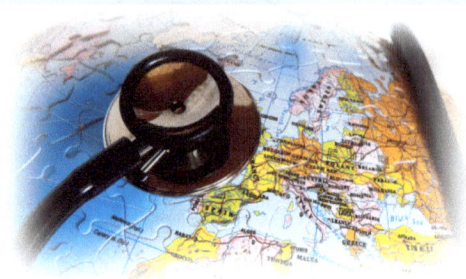

Vitiligo

1) Chronic, depigmenting condition due to unknown cause
2) Sharply demarcated areas of skin become without melanin
3) Most common on the face
4) Topical glucocorticoids and photochemotherapy are used to promote repigmentation with varying degrees of success

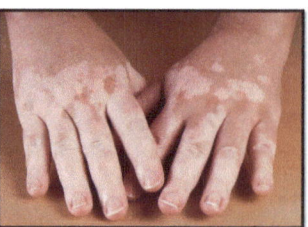

Associated with diabetes mellitus, hypothyroidism, pernicious anemia, and Addison disease

22 | Impetigo

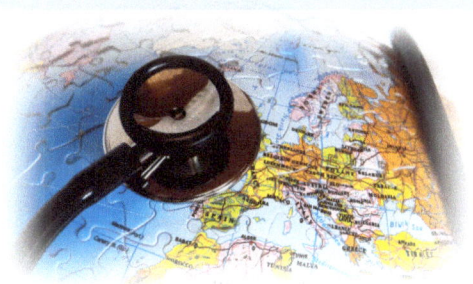

Impetigo

Impetigo
1) Contagious skin infection most commonly found in children
2) most commonly caused by Staphylococcus aureus
3) Clinical features include facial pruritus - yellow crusted lesions around mucocutaneous surfaces - erythematous vesicles (blisters)
4) Treatment by Topical antibiotics (*Mupirocin*)

Use Oral antibiotics if severe
Use Dicloxacillin or Cephalexin in outbreaks

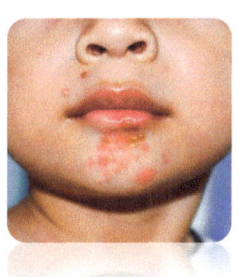

23 Skin Abscess

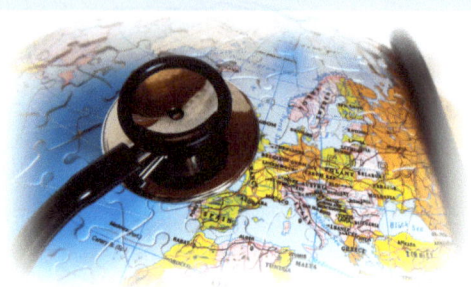

Skin Abscess

Skin Abscess
1) Subcutaneous collection of pus most commonly caused by staphylococcal bacteria, usually MRSA.
2) Erythematous, fluctuant, and localized swelling in skin
3) Tender on palpation
4) Can occur as collection of multiple infected hair follicles (Carbuncle)
5) Treatment is drainage + antibiotics (such as co-trimoxazole, that cover MRSA)

Note: Facial abscess can lead to cavernous sinus thrombosis (CVST)

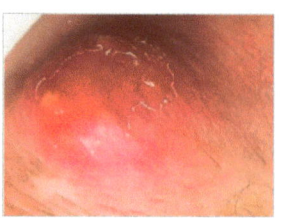

24 Cellulitis

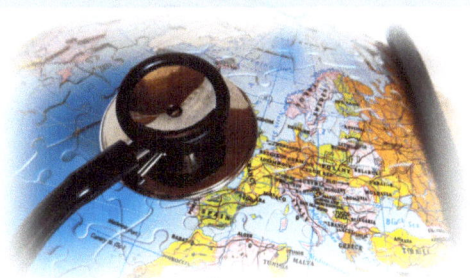

Cellulitis

Cellulitis
Cellulitis is an acute bacterial infection of the dermis and subcutaneous tissue.
It is most commonly caused by group A streptococci

Risk factors include:
Intravenous (IV) drug use, Diabetes mellitus (DM), Immunocompromise, Penetration of skin (skin ulcer, surgery, trauma), Previous cellulitis, Venous or lymphatic dysfunction

Cellulitis

Cellulitis

Manifestations include erythema, swollen and painful skin, myalgias, chills; warmth in involved area, fever

It may occur near a wound

Associated with increased white blood cell count (WBC), erythrocyte sedimentation rate (ESR), and high C-reactive protein (CRP)

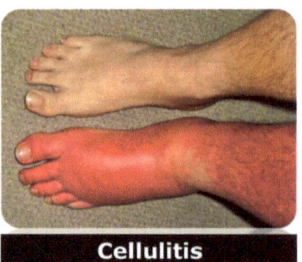

Cellulitis

Skin and wound cultures are rarely useful in cellulitis because they frequently contain other normal skin flora or high false negative results.

Cellulitis

Cellulitis

Treatment

1) Oral cephalosporins or penicillinase-resistant β-lactams for 10 to 14 days
2) IV antibiotics for severe cases or bacteremia

Patients with pus in the lesion or at high risk for MRSA should receive Co-trimoxazole or Linezolid or IV Vancomycin.

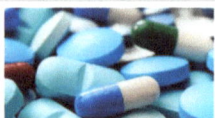

Complications include abscess, sepsis, necrotizing fasciitis
Recurrence rate is as high as 20-50%.

25 Necrotizing Fasciitis

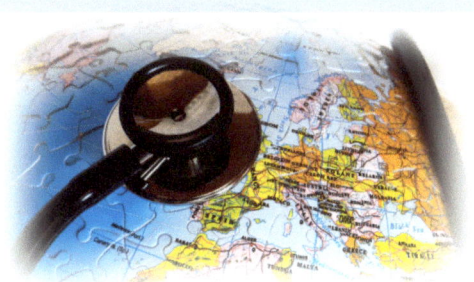

Necrotizing Fasciitis

Necrotizing Fasciitis
1) Quickly spreading group polymicrobial infection of fascial planes leading to extensive soft tissue destruction and systemic infection
2) Erythematous, warm, and swollen skin
3) Loss of sensation in involved tissue
4) Fever, crepitus,
5) Purple discoloration + bullae.

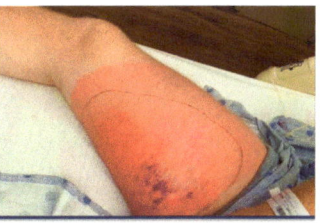

Characterized by pain out of proportion of examination.

26 Warts

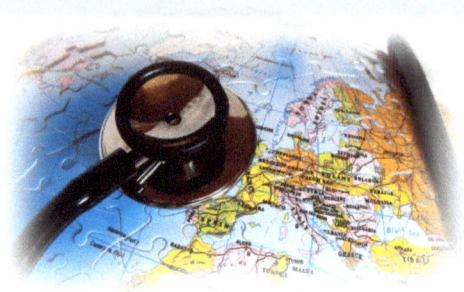

Warts

Warts are caused by HPV and are transmitted via skin-to-skin contact. (For genital warts, transmission is via intimate sexual contact).

Most warts disappear spontaneously within 1 to 2 years. However, if the condition is left untreated, more warts can appear.

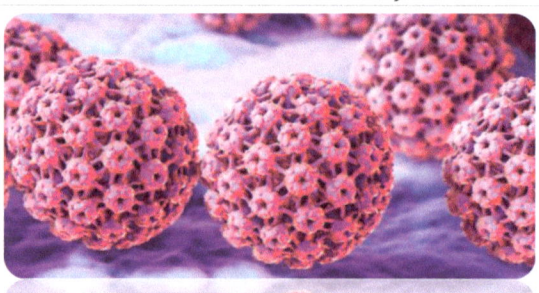

Warts

Types

The common wart (Verruca vulgaris)—most common type. May occur anywhere, but the most common sites include elbows, knees, fingers, and palms. Appearance: flesh-colored or whitish with a hyperkeratotic surface.

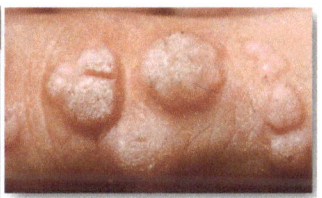

Warts

Types

The flat wart (**Verruca plana**). Common sites include the chin/face, dorsum of hands, and legs. Appears flesh-colored with smooth papules and a flat surface.

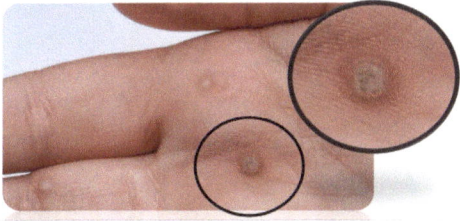

Warts

Types

The plantar wart (Verruca plantaris). Solitary or multiple warts found on the plantar side of the foot; can cause foot pain if located on pressure areas (e.g., metatarsal head, heel).
Appearance: flesh colored with a rough, hyperkeratotic surface.

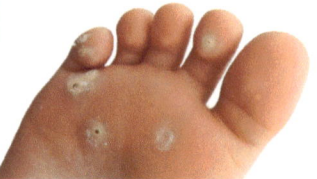

Warts

Types

Anogenital wart (**Condyloma acuminatum**).
Condyloma acuminatum is the most common STD
Commonly associated with HPV 6 and 11. The warts are papillary or cauliflower-like

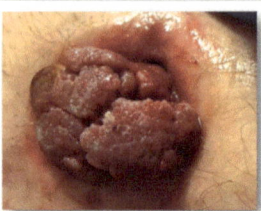

Condyloma acuminatum appears as single or multiple soft, fleshy growths on the genitalia, perineum, and anus.

HPV (types 16, 18) infection can lead to cervical cancer in women (Pap smear is important), and protective vaccines are available.

Warts

Treatment of warts
First line is typically salicylic acid or cryotherapy (freezing with liquid nitrogen).

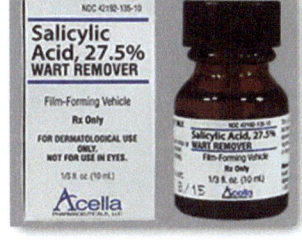

For refractory warts, options include 5-FU, intralesional bleomycin, topical or intralesional immunotherapy (Candida antigen), surgical therapy, laser therapy, imiquimod, and many others.

27 Molluscum Contagiosum

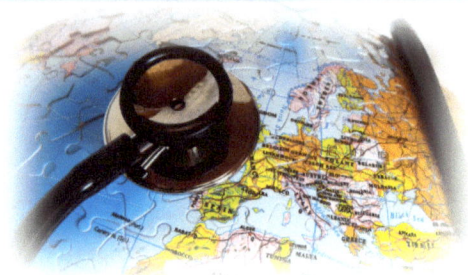

Molluscum Contagiosum

1) A common, self-limited viral infection caused by a **poxvirus**
2) Common in sexually active young adults and in children.
3) It manifests as asymptomatic small umbilicated papules (2 to 5 mm)
4) It is transmitted via skin-to-skin contact

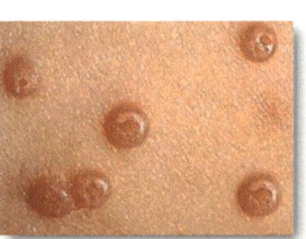

Note (1): Sexual contact can lead to genital involvement and is highly contagious.
Note (2): In HIV-positive patients, lesions can be extensive.

Molluscum Contagiosum

Often regresses spontaneously, but multiple treatment modalities are effective (such as Curettage, drops containing podophyllin and cantharidin, cryosurgery)

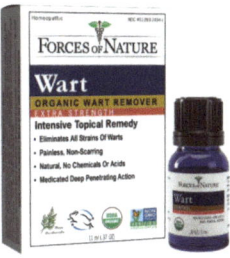

Note: Molluscum Contagiosum may leave a scar

28 | Herpes Zoster (Shingles)

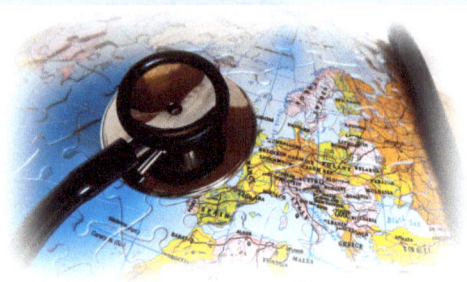

Herpes Zoster (Shingles)

Caused by **reactivation** of the varicella-zoster virus, which remains dormant in the dorsal root ganglia and is reactivated in times of stress, infection, or illness.
It is not as contagious as chickenpox.

Shingles only occurs in those who have previously had chickenpox.

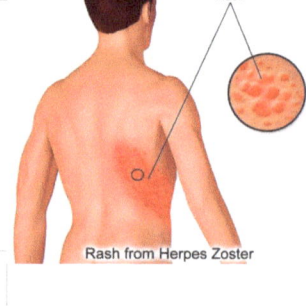

Rash from Herpes Zoster

Herpes Zoster (Shingles)

It is typically seen in patients above 50 years of age.

If occurred in patients less than 50 years of age you should suspect an immunosuppressed state.

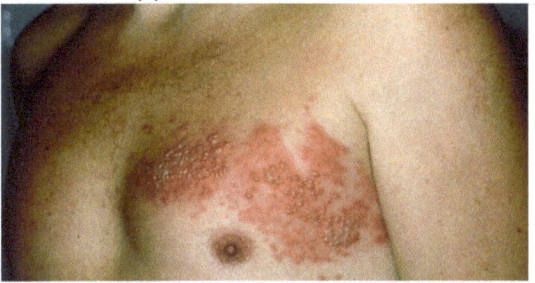

Herpes Zoster (Shingles)

Clinical Features
1) Severe pain and rash in a dermatomal distribution.
2) Pain comes before the rash.
3) Rash is characterized by grouped vesicles on an erythematous base.
4) If severe, low-grade fever and malaise may be present.
5) The most common sites of involvement are the thorax (most cases) and trigeminal distribution (especially ophthalmic division).

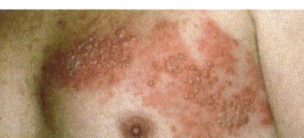

Affected sites ma also include other cranial nerves, as well as arms and legs.

Herpes Zoster (Shingles)

Complications of Herpes Zoster
1) Postherpetic neuralgia
Manifests as excruciating pain that persists after the lesions have cleared, and does not respond to analgesics
Can be chronic and debilitating
2) Uveitis
3) Dissemination
4) Meningoencephalitis
5) Deafness

Herpes Zoster (Shingles)

Treatment
1) Keep the lesions clean and dry.
2) **Analgesics** for pain relief (Aspirin or acetaminophen; codeine if needed).
3) **Antiviral agents** (acyclovir, famciclovir, valacyclovir) to reduce the pain, decrease the length of illness, and reduce the risk of postherpetic neuralgia.

In severe cases, administer a local injection of triamcinolone in lidocaine.

The use of corticosteroids to decrease the incidence of postherpetic neuralgia remains controversial.

Herpes Zoster (Shingles)

Treatment
Live vaccine has been shown to be effective in reducing the number of cases of shingles in patients over the age of 60 in addition to reducing the severity and duration of postherpetic neuralgia in patients who do end up with the disease. The vaccine should be recommended to all patients over 60 who do not have contraindications.

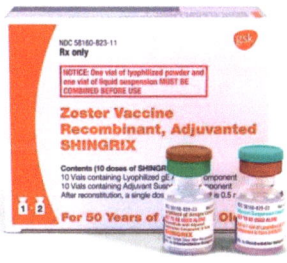

29 Dermatophytes

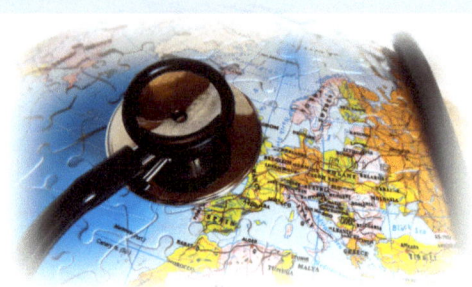

Dermatophytes

Dermatophytes are superficial fungi that infect cutaneous epithelium, nails, and hair.
The three main genera of dermatophytes are Trichophyton, Microsporum, and Epidermophyton.

Treat tinea capitis and onychomycosis with oral antifungal agents. Others are treated with topical antifungals.

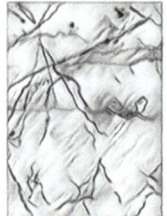 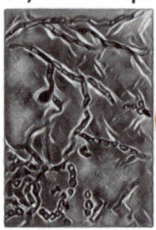

Scrape lesions and use KOH preparation to visualize the fungus.

Dermatophytes
Tinea Corporis (Ringworm)
❶ More common on Body and Trunk
❷ All ages
❸ Pinkish annular lesions
❹ Direct microscopy: Hyphae from skin scrapings with KOH preparation
❺ Topical antifungals (e.g. Ketoconazole and Miconazole)

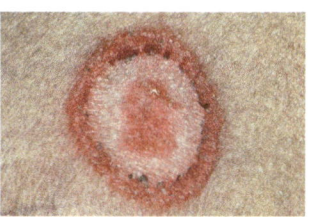

Dermatophytes
Tinea Capitis
❶ Scalp
❷ More common in Children
❸ Areas of scaling with hair loss
❹ ?! Pruritus
❹ Direct microscopy:
Hair fluorescence
Present: Microsporum spp.
Absent: Trichophyton spp.
❺ Treat with ORAL griseofulvin (antifungal)

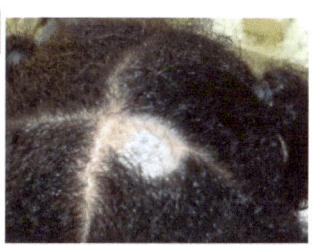

Dermatophytes
Tinea pedis (athlete's foot)
❶ Feet- Web spaces of toes
❷ Young adults
❸ Scaling-Erythema-Pruritus
❹ Direct microscopy: Hyphae from skin scrapings with KOH preparation
❺ Use topical antifungals (e.g., Ketoconazole and Miconazole) PLUS good foot hygiene

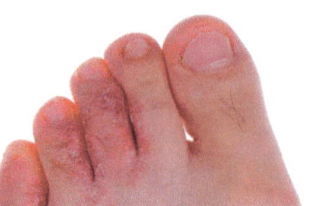

Dermatophytes
Tinea cruris (Jock itch)
❶ More common on Groin & Inner thighs
❷ Adults (Males> Females))
❸ Scaling & Erythema
❹ Direct microscopy:
❺ Topical antifungals (e.g. Ketoconazole and Miconazole) and good hygiene.

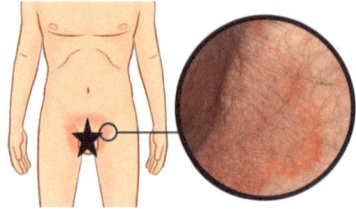

Dermatophytes
Tinea unguium (Onychomycosis)
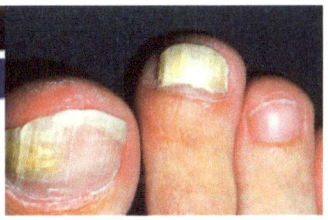
1. Nails
2. Elderly people
3. Thick opacified nails
4. Direct microscopy: (Nail scrapings)
5. ORAL griseofulvin (antifungal)

30 Tinea Versicolor

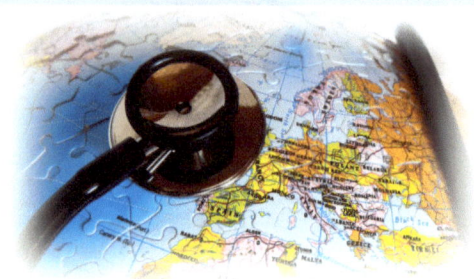

Tinea Versicolor

1) A common superficial fungal infection likely caused by several species in the **Malassezia group** (part of the normal skin flora)
2) Characteristic lesions are well demarcated and most commonly affect the trunk.
3) Lesions may be hyper- or hypopigmented and can range in color from brown to tan to white.
4) Adolescents and young adults are most commonly affected.

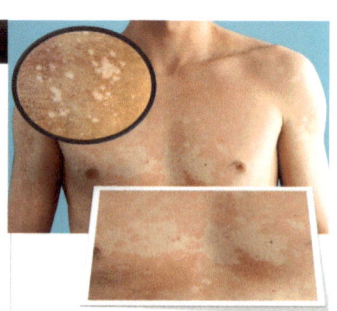

Tinea Versicolor

Diagnosis should be made with KOH prep, which will show the "spaghetti and meatballs" pattern consistent with both hyphae and yeast balls.

Hot/humid weather, excessive sweating, and skin oils may contribute to transformation from normal skin flora to pathologic condition.

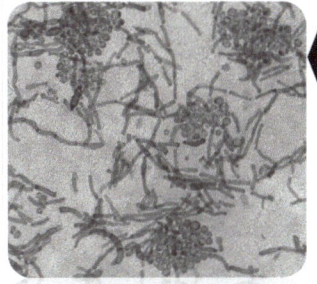

Spaghetti and Meatballs (**KOH**)

Tinea Versicolor

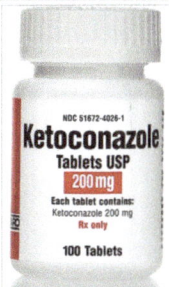

(1) Treatment consists of oral or topical **antifungals**, depending on the severity of the disease. **(2) Selenium sulfide** lotion may also be helpful.

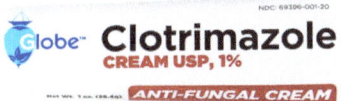

31 Scabies

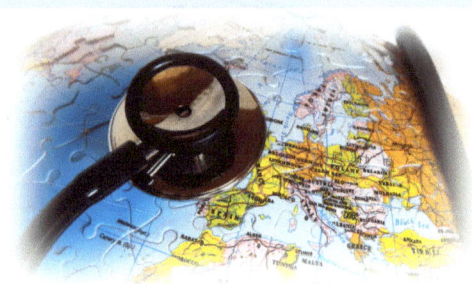

Scabies

1) Caused by the human skin **mite** Sarcoptes scabiei.
2) Highly contagious—transmitted via skin-to-skin contact or through towels, bed linens, or clothes.

Pathogenesis: The mite tunnels into the epidermis, lay eggs, and deposit feces (called scybala). A delayed type IV hypersensitivity reaction develops toward the mites, eggs, and feces, causing intense pruritus.

The head, neck, palms, and soles are typically spared.

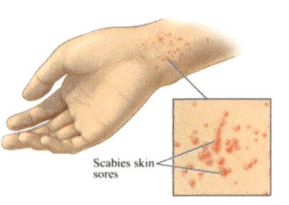

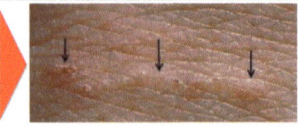

Scabies

1) **Severe pruritus**—Most severe during the night.
2) Burrows—linear marks (several millimeters in length) represent the tunneled path of the mite.
3) Scratching may lead to excoriations.
4) Eczematous plaques, crusted papules, or secondary bacterial

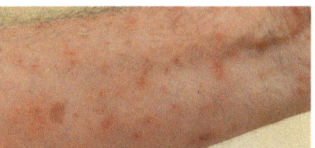

Suspect scabies in any patient who has persistent, generalized, severe pruritus.

Common locations include the fingers, interdigital areas, and wrists.

Scabies

Diagnosis
1) Look for characteristic **burrows** on hands, wrists, and ankles, and in the genital region.
2) Confirm the diagnosis by scraping the burrow with a scalpel and examining it under a **microscope** to detect the presence of mites, ova, or scybala.

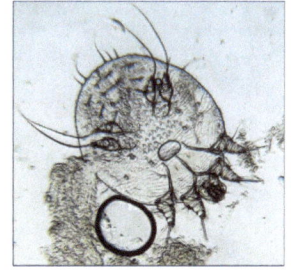

Scabies

Treatment
Specific medications.
1) **Permethrin** 5% cream is often used as first-line treatment
2) Should be applied to every area of the body (head to toe)
3) Patients should leave cream on overnight (>8 to 10 hours) and wash it off the next morning.

Other options include oral ivermectin or topical lindane (γ-benzene-hexachloride).

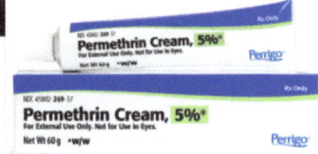

Scabies

General recommendations.
Treat all close contacts of the patient simultaneously (even if asymptomatic) with Permethrin 5% cream.

Instruct the patient to thoroughly wash all underwear and bed linens.

Pruritus may continue for a few weeks after treatment as dead mites are shed from the skin. Use topical corticosteroids and oral antihistamines to control pruritus during this time.

32 Actinic Keratosis

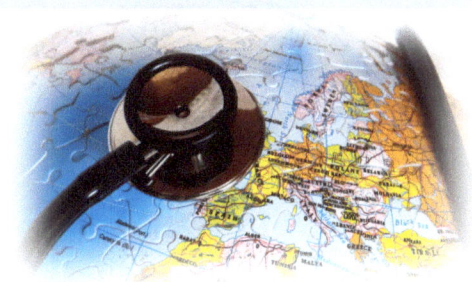

Actinic Keratosis
(Also Called Solar Keratosis)

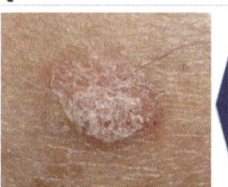 Small, rough, scaly lesions due to prolonged and repeated sun exposure.

Most commonly seen in fair-skinned people.
Lesions are typically seen on the face.

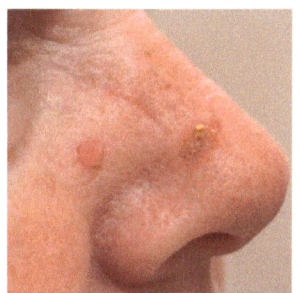

Actinic Keratosis

(Also Called Solar Keratosis)
The risk of malignant transformation is low (1 in 1,000),
Biopsy is still recommended for the lesions to exclude SCC.
Additionally, lesions which become indurated, tender, or bleed spontaneously must be biopsied to exclude SCC.

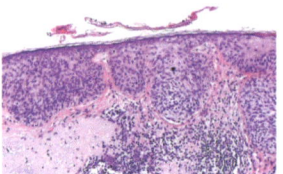

Actinic Keratosis

(Also Called Solar Keratosis)
Treatment options include surgical removal (scraping), freezing with liquid nitrogen, or application of topical 5-FU for multiple lesions (destroys sun-damaged skin cells).

Prevention: advise patients to avoid excessive sun exposure and to use sunscreen.

33 Seborrheic Keratosis

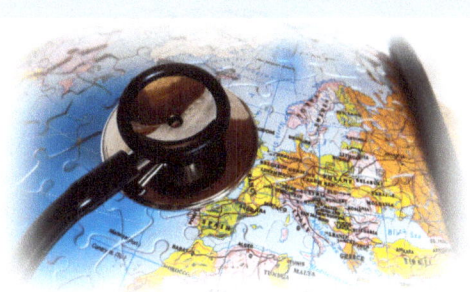

Seborrheic Keratosis

Seborrheic Keratosis

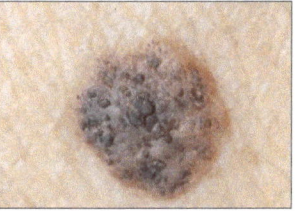

1) These are very common skin lesions that begin to appear after the age of 30 years (?! autosomal dominant).
2) They can be located anywhere but are more common on the face and trunk.
3) They are harmless growths with no malignant potential.
4) There is no association with sunlight.

Seborrheic Keratosis

Seborrheic Keratosis
They are slightly elevated plaques, gradually turning darker in color, and appear as if they were "stuck" on the skin.

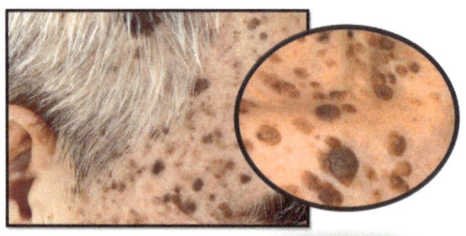

Seborrheic Keratosis

Seborrheic Keratosis
Treatment is not necessary and is only for cosmetic reasons: **Liquid nitrogen cryotherapy** or curettage is effective and easily performed in the office setting.

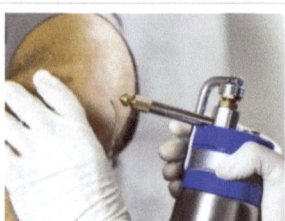

34 Keratoacanthoma

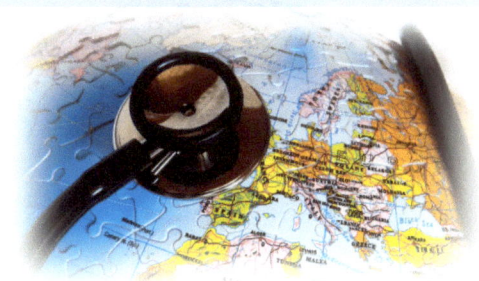

Keratoacanthoma

Epithelial tumors which clinically resemble squamous cell carcinoma (SCC).
The **lesions** progress to the typical dome with central crater containing keratinous material over the course of several weeks.
(**Note:** This type of growth is very rare for SCC).
Treatment involves observation, as many of these will regress spontaneously over several months.

Keratoacanthoma

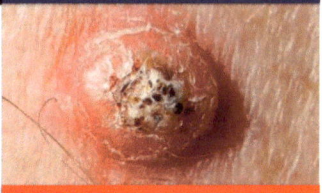

Lesions grow VERY quickly.

Basal Cell Carcinoma (BCC)

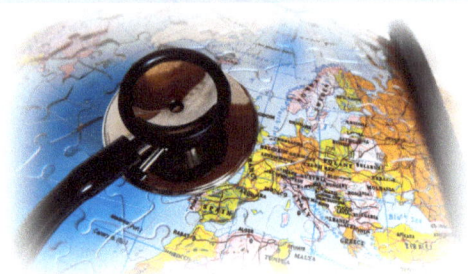

Basal Cell Carcinoma (BCC)

1) Basal cell carcinoma (BCC) is the most common skin cancer (60-75% of all skin cancers).
2) Most frequently in fair-skinned individuals who burn easily and involves sun-exposed areas (most important risk factor), such as the head and neck (**Note:** the nose is the most common site).
3) Surgical resection is curative.
4) Metastasis is extremely rare but can be locally destructive.

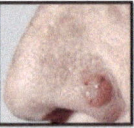 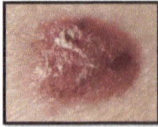

A pearly, smooth papule with rolled edges and surface telangiectases

36 Squamous Cell Carcinoma (SCC)

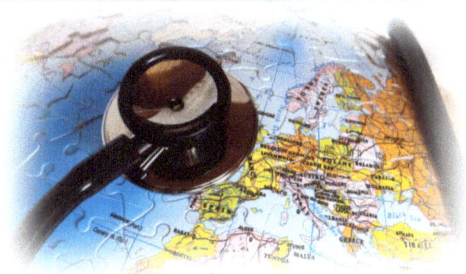

Squamous Cell Carcinoma

1) Sunlight exposure is the most important risk factor for SCC.
2) Appears as a crusting, ulcerated nodule or erosion
3) The possibility of metastasis is higher than with BCC, but much lower than with melanoma.
4) Prognosis is excellent if it is completely excised (95% cure rate).

Concomitant actinic keratoses, chronic skin damage, and immunosuppressive therapy are also risk factors.

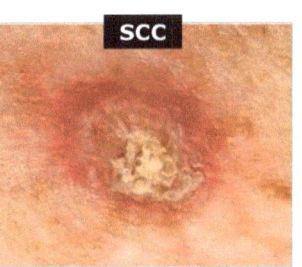

37 Melanoma

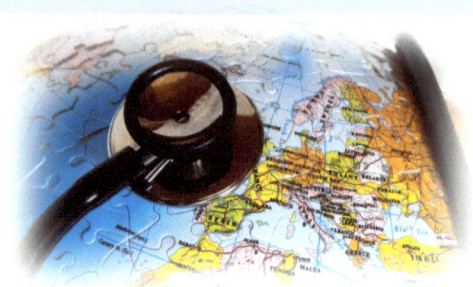

Melanoma

Most aggressive form of skin cancer and the number one cause of death due to skin cancer.
Increasing incidence worldwide

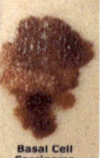
Basal Cell Carcinoma

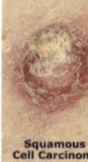
Squamous Cell Carcinoma

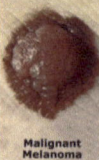
Malignant Melanoma

Risk Factors:
Fair complexion
Numerous moles
Sun exposure
Family history of melanoma
Xeroderma pigmentosa)
Increasing age

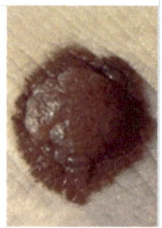

Melanoma

Large numbers of nevi (moles)
Although most melanomas arise de novo, they may arise from pre-existing nevi in up to 50% of cases. Any change in a nevus is concerning because it may indicate malignancy or malignant transformation.

Changes in a mole that suggest malignancy include:
1) Change in color
2) Bleeding
3) Ulceration
4) A Papule arising from the center of an existing nevus

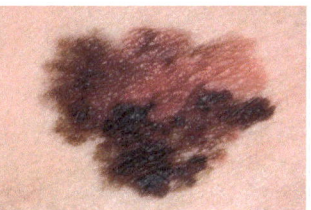

Melanoma

Rule for the early detection of melanoma

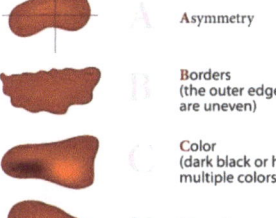

Asymmetry

Borders
(the outer edges are uneven)

Color
(dark black or have multiple colors)

Diameter
(greater than 6 mm)

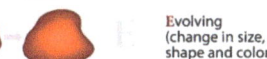

Evolving
(change in size, shape and color)

Melanoma
Dysplastic nevus syndrome
Numerous, atypical moles—these tend to be large with indistinct borders and variations in color. The chances of a single dysplastic nevus becoming a melanoma are small
If dysplastic nevus syndrome and a family history of melanoma are present, the risk of developing melanoma approaches 100%
Prophylactic excision is recommended

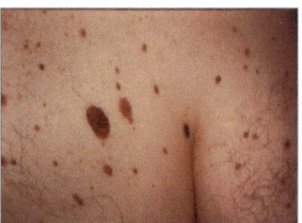

Melanoma
Growth phases
1) Radial (initial) growth phase
Growth is predominantly lateral within the epidermis
There is a good prognosis with surgical resection because metastasis is unlikely

Melanoma
Growth phases

2) Vertical (later) phase
Growth extends into the reticular dermis or beyond
Lymphatic or hematogenous metastasis may occur

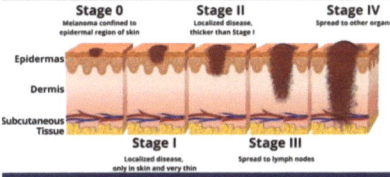

Depth of invasion is the most important indicator of prognosis

Melanoma
Clinical Features

Melanoma may present with some or all of the following features:
Asymmetry
Border irregularity
Color variegation—ranging from pink to blue to black
Diameter greater than 6 mm
Evolution—changes in size, shape, or color

Melanoma

Diagnosis
Excisional biopsy is the standard of care for diagnosis of any suspicious skin lesion.

Early detection is the most important way to prevent death, because prognosis is directly related to depth of invasion.

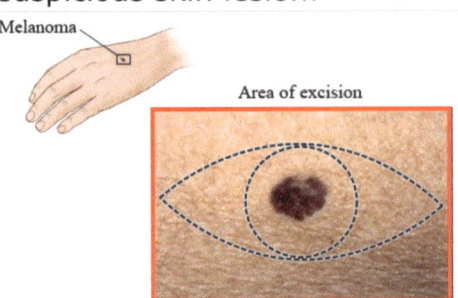

www.ingramcontent.com/pod-product-compliance
Lightning Source LLC
Chambersburg PA
CBHW040222220526
45473CB00001B/87